DR. BARBARA CURE FOR HIGH BLOOD PRESSURE

Discover powerful and natural remedies to effectively treat and cure high blood pressure for your well-being and vitality

Odesa Mulan

Table of Contents

COPYRIGHT © 2023

CHAPTER ONE

Understanding High Blood Pressure: Causes, Risks, and Complications

High blood pressure, medically known as hypertension, is a common yet potentially serious condition that affects millions of people worldwide. It's often referred to as a "silent killer" because it usually has no symptoms but can lead to severe health complications if left untreated. Understanding the causes, risks, and complications associated with high blood pressure is crucial for effective management and prevention.

Causes of High Blood Pressure

High blood pressure can have various causes, both modifiable and non-modifiable. One of the primary factors contributing to hypertension is lifestyle choices. Poor diet, high in salt, saturated fats, and cholesterol, along with low intake of fruits and vegetables, can increase blood pressure. Additionally, lack of physical activity and excess weight or obesity are significant contributors to hypertension.

Genetics also play a significant role in the development of high blood pressure. Individuals with a family history of hypertension are at a higher risk of developing the condition themselves. Genetic factors can influence how the body regulates blood pressure, making some individuals more susceptible to hypertension than others.

Other underlying health conditions can also lead to high blood pressure. These include:

1. **Kidney Disease**: The kidneys play a crucial role in regulating blood pressure by controlling fluid balance and filtering waste from the blood. Dysfunction in the kidneys can disrupt this process, leading to hypertension.

2. **Endocrine Disorders**: Hormonal imbalances, such as those seen in conditions like hyperthyroidism or Cushing's syndrome, can contribute to high blood pressure.

3. **Obstructive Sleep Apnea**: This sleep disorder is characterized by pauses in breathing during sleep, leading to oxygen deprivation and increased blood pressure.

4. **Adrenal Gland Tumors**: Tumors of the adrenal glands can produce excess hormones that raise blood pressure.

5. **Certain Medications**: Some medications, such as nonsteroidal anti-inflammatory drugs (NSAIDs), decongestants, and oral contraceptives, can elevate blood pressure in some individuals.

Identifying the specific cause of high blood pressure in an individual is essential for determining the most appropriate treatment and management plan.

Risks Associated with High Blood Pressure

High blood pressure is a significant risk factor for various health complications, including cardiovascular disease, stroke, kidney disease, and vision loss. When blood pressure remains consistently elevated, it can damage the arteries and organs throughout the body over time, leading to serious health consequences.

1. **Cardiovascular Disease**: Hypertension is a leading cause of heart disease, including coronary artery disease, heart attacks, and heart failure. Elevated blood pressure puts increased strain on the heart, leading to thickening and narrowing of the arteries, reduced blood flow to the heart muscle, and an increased risk of heart attacks and other cardiovascular events.

2. **Stroke**: High blood pressure is the most important modifiable risk factor for stroke, a potentially life-threatening condition caused by a disruption of blood flow to the brain. Uncontrolled hypertension can lead to the formation of blood clots or the rupture of blood vessels in the brain, resulting in a stroke.

3. **Kidney Disease**: Chronic hypertension can damage the blood vessels in the kidneys, impairing their ability to filter waste from the blood effectively. Over time, this can lead to kidney

disease or kidney failure, requiring dialysis or transplantation.

4. **Vision Problems**: Hypertension can damage the blood vessels in the eyes, leading to vision problems or even blindness. Conditions such as hypertensive retinopathy and optic nerve damage can result from uncontrolled high blood pressure.

5. **Peripheral Artery Disease (PAD)**: Elevated blood pressure can cause narrowing and hardening of the arteries in the legs and arms, reducing blood flow to these extremities. This can lead to symptoms such as leg pain, numbness, and poor wound healing, and increase the risk of infections and tissue damage.

Complications of High Blood Pressure

The complications of high blood pressure can significantly impact an individual's quality of life and may require intensive medical intervention to manage effectively.

1. **Heart Failure**: Chronic hypertension can weaken the heart muscle over time, leading to heart failure. This condition occurs when the heart is unable to pump enough blood to meet the body's needs, resulting in symptoms such as fatigue, shortness of breath, and fluid retention.

2. **Aneurysm**: High blood pressure can contribute to the formation of aneurysms, which are weakened areas in the walls of blood vessels that can balloon out and potentially rupture. A ruptured aneurysm is a life-threatening medical emergency that requires immediate treatment.

3. **Cognitive Decline**: There is growing evidence to suggest that uncontrolled hypertension may contribute to cognitive decline and an increased risk of dementia, including Alzheimer's disease. Elevated blood pressure can damage the small blood vessels in the brain, leading to reduced blood flow and oxygen delivery to brain cells.

4. **Sexual Dysfunction**: High blood pressure can affect sexual function in both men and women. In men, hypertension can lead to erectile dysfunction by impairing blood flow to the penis. In women, it can reduce arousal and lubrication, making sexual activity less enjoyable.

5. **Pregnancy Complications**: Hypertension during pregnancy, such as preeclampsia or gestational hypertension, can pose serious risks to both the mother and the baby. These complications may include preterm birth, low birth weight, and maternal complications such as seizures and organ damage.

Conclusion

High blood pressure is a common yet serious medical condition that requires careful management to prevent complications and improve long-term health outcomes. Understanding the causes, risks, and complications associated with hypertension is essential for effective prevention, diagnosis, and treatment. Lifestyle modifications, including a healthy diet, regular exercise, stress management, and medication when necessary, are crucial components of managing high blood pressure and reducing the risk of associated complications. Regular monitoring of blood pressure and timely intervention are key to maintaining optimal health and well-being.

CHAPTER TWO

Meet Dr. Barbara: Her Background and Expertise in Herbal Medicine

Dr. Barbara is a renowned herbalist with a deep passion for natural healing and a wealth of expertise in herbal medicine. Her journey into the world of herbalism began early in life, influenced by her upbringing in a family that valued traditional healing practices. From a young age, she was fascinated by the power of plants to promote health and well-being, which set her on a path of exploration and discovery in the field of herbal medicine.

Background and Education

Dr. Barbara's academic journey laid the foundation for her career in herbal medicine. She pursued a Bachelor of Science degree in Botany, where she developed a profound understanding of plant biology, ecology, and pharmacology. This educational background provided her with a solid scientific framework for studying the medicinal properties of plants and understanding how they interact with the human body.

Driven by her passion for herbalism, Dr. Barbara furthered her studies by obtaining a Master of Science degree in Herbal Medicine. During this time, she delved deep into the principles of traditional herbal medicine systems from around the world, including Traditional Chinese Medicine (TCM), Ayurveda, and

Western herbalism. She studied the therapeutic properties of hundreds of medicinal plants, learning how to identify, cultivate, and prepare them for therapeutic use.

In addition to her formal education, Dr. Barbara embarked on extensive fieldwork and apprenticeships with master herbalists, indigenous healers, and botanical experts. These immersive experiences allowed her to learn directly from practitioners who passed down traditional knowledge and wisdom through generations, enriching her understanding of herbal medicine beyond textbooks and classrooms.

Expertise in Herbal Medicine

Dr. Barbara's expertise in herbal medicine spans a wide range of areas, including herbal materia medica, formulation, clinical practice, and research. She is deeply knowledgeable about the therapeutic properties of medicinal plants and their applications in addressing various health concerns.

1. **Herbal Materia Medica**: Dr. Barbara has an extensive knowledge of medicinal plants, including their botanical characteristics, phytochemical composition, and traditional uses. She understands the importance of sourcing high-quality herbs and maintains a comprehensive materia medica that serves as a valuable reference in her practice.

2. **Formulation**: Drawing on her understanding of herbal energetics and therapeutic actions, Dr. Barbara excels in

formulating customized herbal remedies to address individual health needs. Whether creating tinctures, teas, capsules, or topical preparations, she carefully selects herbs and adjusts dosages to optimize efficacy and safety.

3. **Clinical Practice**: With years of clinical experience, Dr. Barbara has successfully helped numerous clients achieve better health outcomes through herbal medicine. She takes a holistic approach to healthcare, considering not only the presenting symptoms but also the underlying imbalances and constitutional factors that contribute to illness.

4. **Research**: Dr. Barbara is actively engaged in herbal medicine research, contributing to the growing body of scientific evidence supporting the efficacy and safety of herbal therapies. She collaborates with fellow researchers and healthcare professionals to design studies, conduct trials, and disseminate findings that contribute to the advancement of herbal medicine as a respected healing modality.

Philosophy and Approach

At the core of Dr. Barbara's practice is a deep respect for nature's wisdom and a belief in the body's innate ability to heal itself when provided with the right support. She views herbal medicine as a holistic approach to wellness that addresses the root causes of illness while promoting balance and harmony within the body.

Dr. Barbara's approach to patient care is compassionate, individualized, and empowering. She takes the time to listen to her clients, understand their unique health challenges, and co-create treatment plans that resonate with their goals and values. She educates and empowers her clients to take an active role in their health journey, providing them with the knowledge and tools they need to make informed decisions about their well-being.

In all her endeavors, Dr. Barbara is guided by a commitment to integrity, excellence, and ethical practice. She upholds rigorous standards of professionalism and continuously seeks to expand her knowledge and skills through ongoing education and collaboration within the herbal medicine community.

Conclusion

Dr. Barbara's background and expertise in herbal medicine are a testament to her dedication to the art and science of natural healing. With a solid foundation in botany, extensive training in herbalism, and years of clinical experience, she brings a wealth of knowledge and wisdom to her practice. Dr. Barbara is passionate about empowering individuals to reclaim their health and vitality through the transformative power of plants, embodying the timeless tradition of herbal medicine in the modern world.

CHAPTER THREE

The Role of Herbs in Blood Pressure Management: Exploring Natural Solutions

High blood pressure, or hypertension, is a common condition that affects millions of people worldwide and is a significant risk factor for cardiovascular disease and other health complications. While conventional treatments such as medications and lifestyle modifications play a crucial role in managing blood pressure, there is growing interest in the potential of herbal medicine as a complementary approach. In this discussion, we will explore the role of herbs in blood pressure management, including their mechanisms of action, evidence-based benefits, and considerations for use.

Mechanisms of Action

Herbs exert their effects on blood pressure through various mechanisms, including:

1. **Vasodilation**: Some herbs have vasodilatory effects, meaning they help widen blood vessels, which can lead to a decrease in blood pressure. This effect is often attributed to compounds such as flavonoids, polyphenols, and nitric oxide precursors found in certain herbs.

2. **Diuretic Action**: Certain herbs possess diuretic properties, promoting the excretion of excess sodium and water from

the body through urine. By reducing fluid volume, these herbs may help lower blood pressure, particularly in individuals with fluid retention.

3. **Antioxidant Activity**: Oxidative stress is implicated in the development and progression of hypertension. Herbs rich in antioxidants, such as flavonoids, vitamin C, and vitamin E, can help neutralize free radicals and protect blood vessels from damage, thereby supporting cardiovascular health.

4. **Anti-inflammatory Effects**: Chronic inflammation is associated with hypertension and cardiovascular disease. Some herbs exhibit anti-inflammatory properties, which may help reduce inflammation and lower blood pressure.

Evidence-Based Benefits

Several herbs have been studied for their potential benefits in blood pressure management. While research is ongoing, some herbs have demonstrated promising results in clinical trials:

1. **Hawthorn (Crataegus spp.)**: Hawthorn is a well-known herb traditionally used for cardiovascular health. Studies suggest that hawthorn extracts may help lower blood pressure by improving blood flow, reducing peripheral resistance, and enhancing cardiac function.

2. **Garlic (Allium sativum)**: Garlic has been shown to have hypotensive effects in both animal and human studies. It

may help lower blood pressure by promoting vasodilation, inhibiting angiotensin-converting enzyme (ACE), and reducing oxidative stress.

3. **Hibiscus (Hibiscus sabdariffa)**: Hibiscus tea has gained attention for its potential antihypertensive effects. Clinical trials have found that hibiscus consumption can lead to significant reductions in systolic and diastolic blood pressure, possibly due to its diuretic and vasodilatory properties.

4. **Olive Leaf (Olea europaea)**: Olive leaf extract contains compounds such as oleuropein, which have been shown to have antihypertensive effects in animal studies. Human studies have reported reductions in blood pressure with olive leaf extract supplementation, although further research is needed.

5. **Astragalus (Astragalus membranaceus)**: Astragalus is an herb used in traditional Chinese medicine for its cardiovascular benefits. Preliminary studies suggest that astragalus may help lower blood pressure by improving endothelial function and reducing oxidative stress.

Considerations for Use

While herbs can be valuable additions to a comprehensive approach to blood pressure management, several considerations should be kept in mind:

1. **Consultation with a Healthcare Provider**: It's essential to consult with a qualified healthcare provider before using herbs for blood pressure management, especially if you're already taking medications or have underlying health conditions. Some herbs may interact with medications or exacerbate certain health conditions.

2. **Quality and Standardization**: When selecting herbal products, opt for reputable brands that adhere to quality standards and provide standardized extracts. This ensures consistency in dosage and potency, enhancing safety and efficacy.

3. **Individualized Approach**: Herbal therapy should be individualized based on factors such as the underlying cause of hypertension, overall health status, and lifestyle factors. A qualified herbalist or healthcare provider can help tailor a treatment plan to meet your specific needs.

4. **Monitoring and Evaluation**: Regular monitoring of blood pressure levels is essential when using herbal therapy for hypertension. Keep track of your blood pressure readings and report any significant changes to your healthcare provider.

5. **Integration with Conventional Treatment**: Herbal medicine should complement, not replace, conventional treatments for hypertension. It's important to continue any prescribed

medications and follow recommended lifestyle modifications while incorporating herbs into your regimen.

Conclusion

Herbal medicine offers a rich array of potential options for blood pressure management, with herbs such as hawthorn, garlic, hibiscus, olive leaf, and astragalus showing promise in clinical research. By understanding the mechanisms of action, evidence-based benefits, and considerations for use, individuals can make informed decisions about integrating herbs into their approach to blood pressure management. However, it's crucial to seek guidance from a qualified healthcare provider to ensure safe and effective use of herbal therapies alongside conventional treatments. With proper guidance and monitoring, herbs can be valuable allies in promoting cardiovascular health and overall well-being.

CHAPTER FOUR

Getting Started: Preparing Mentally and Physically for Herbal Treatment

Embarking on a journey of herbal treatment requires careful preparation, both mentally and physically, to optimize the effectiveness and safety of the therapeutic process. Whether you're seeking herbal remedies for a specific health concern or simply aiming to enhance your overall well-being, taking proactive steps to prepare yourself can set the stage for a successful and fulfilling experience. In this guide, we'll explore strategies for preparing mentally and physically for herbal treatment to maximize its benefits and ensure a positive outcome.

Mental Preparation

1. **Set Clear Intentions**: Before starting herbal treatment, take some time to reflect on your goals and intentions. What specific health concerns are you hoping to address? What outcomes are you aiming to achieve? Setting clear intentions can help focus your efforts and guide your journey toward wellness.

2. **Cultivate a Positive Mindset**: Approach herbal treatment with an open mind and a positive attitude. Believe in the potential of herbs to support your health and well-being, and

trust in your body's innate ability to heal. Cultivating a positive mindset can enhance your receptivity to herbal remedies and amplify their therapeutic effects.

3. **Educate Yourself**: Knowledge is empowering when it comes to herbal medicine. Take the time to educate yourself about the herbs you'll be using, their therapeutic properties, and any potential risks or contraindications. Understanding how herbs work and what to expect can alleviate anxiety and build confidence in their efficacy.

4. **Manage Expectations**: While herbal medicine can offer profound benefits, it's important to manage your expectations and recognize that healing takes time. Results may not be immediate, and it may require patience and persistence to achieve your desired outcomes. Stay committed to your herbal regimen while remaining realistic about the timeline for progress.

5. **Stay Mindful and Present**: Incorporate mindfulness practices into your daily routine to stay grounded and present throughout your herbal treatment journey. Mindfulness techniques such as meditation, deep breathing, and mindful eating can help reduce stress, enhance self-awareness, and foster a deeper connection with your body's healing process.

Physical Preparation

1. **Assess Your Health**: Before starting herbal treatment, conduct a comprehensive assessment of your health status with the guidance of a qualified healthcare provider. Identify any underlying health conditions, medications, or allergies that may impact your ability to use certain herbs safely. This information will inform your herbal treatment plan and ensure personalized care.

2. **Optimize Your Lifestyle**: Herbal treatment is most effective when combined with a healthy lifestyle that supports overall well-being. Prioritize factors such as nutritious diet, regular exercise, adequate sleep, stress management, and hydration to create a supportive environment for herbal therapy. These lifestyle habits lay the foundation for optimal health and can enhance the effectiveness of herbal remedies.

3. **Gather Necessary Supplies**: Stock up on the herbs and herbal preparations recommended for your treatment plan. Depending on your preferences and the nature of your health concerns, this may include dried herbs for teas, tinctures, capsules, essential oils, or topical preparations. Ensure that you have access to high-quality herbs from reputable sources to maximize their potency and safety.

4. **Create a Healing Environment**: Designate a peaceful and nurturing space in your home where you can engage in

herbal treatments and self-care practices. Surround yourself with elements that promote relaxation and healing, such as soft lighting, calming music, aromatherapy diffusers, and comfortable seating. Cultivate an atmosphere that supports your journey toward wellness.

5. **Establish a Routine**: Incorporate herbal treatment into your daily routine to ensure consistency and adherence. Set aside dedicated time each day for herbal remedies, whether it's brewing a cup of herbal tea, taking herbal supplements, or applying herbal preparations topically. Consistency is key to maximizing the benefits of herbal therapy and achieving sustainable results.

Conclusion

Preparing mentally and physically for herbal treatment is an essential step toward optimizing its effectiveness and ensuring a positive therapeutic experience. By setting clear intentions, cultivating a positive mindset, educating yourself, and staying mindful and present, you can approach herbal medicine with confidence and receptivity. Additionally, assessing your health, optimizing your lifestyle, gathering necessary supplies, creating a healing environment, and establishing a routine will help lay the groundwork for a successful herbal treatment journey. With careful preparation and commitment to holistic wellness, you can harness the healing power of herbs to support your health and vitality.

CHAPTER FIVE

Herbal Remedies for Lowering Blood Pressure: Identifying Effective Plant Compounds

High blood pressure, or hypertension, is a prevalent health concern that increases the risk of cardiovascular disease and other complications. While lifestyle modifications and medications are commonly prescribed for managing blood pressure, many individuals seek natural alternatives, including herbal remedies. Numerous plants contain bioactive compounds with potential hypotensive effects, offering promising avenues for blood pressure management. In this exploration, we'll identify effective plant compounds found in herbal remedies for lowering blood pressure and examine their mechanisms of action and evidence-based benefits.

1. Flavonoids

Flavonoids are a diverse group of polyphenolic compounds found abundantly in fruits, vegetables, and medicinal herbs. Several flavonoids have demonstrated potential antihypertensive effects through various mechanisms:

- **Quercetin**: Found in foods such as apples, onions, and citrus fruits, quercetin has been shown to exert vasodilatory effects, enhance nitric oxide production, and inhibit angiotensin-converting enzyme (ACE), a key regulator of blood pressure.

- **Kaempferol**: Present in foods like broccoli, kale, and tea, kaempferol exhibits antioxidant and anti-inflammatory properties, which may contribute to its blood pressure-lowering effects.

- **Rutin**: Abundant in buckwheat, citrus fruits, and berries, rutin has been studied for its potential to improve endothelial function, reduce oxidative stress, and lower blood pressure.

2. Polyphenols

Polyphenols are another class of bioactive compounds found in various plant-based foods and beverages. Certain polyphenols have been investigated for their hypotensive properties:

- **Resveratrol**: Found in red wine, grapes, and berries, resveratrol has been shown to enhance endothelial function, increase nitric oxide production, and improve blood vessel elasticity, contributing to its blood pressure-lowering effects.

- **Epigallocatechin gallate (EGCG)**: Abundant in green tea, EGCG exhibits antioxidant, anti-inflammatory, and vasodilatory properties, which may help reduce blood pressure levels.

3. Alkaloids

Alkaloids are nitrogen-containing compounds found in various medicinal herbs, some of which possess hypotensive properties:

- **Rauwolfia alkaloids**: Derived from the Rauwolfia serpentina plant, these compounds inhibit the activity of neurotransmitters such as norepinephrine, leading to vasodilation and reduced blood pressure. Rauwolfia alkaloids are used in traditional herbal medicine for hypertension management.

- **Berberine**: Found in plants like goldenseal, barberry, and Oregon grape, berberine has been studied for its potential antihypertensive effects, including vasodilation, inhibition of smooth muscle contraction, and modulation of endothelial function.

4. Terpenoids

Terpenoids are a diverse group of compounds found in essential oils and aromatic plants, some of which exhibit hypotensive effects:

- **Limonene**: Found in citrus fruits and herbs like peppermint and rosemary, limonene has been studied for its potential to lower blood pressure through vasodilation and relaxation of smooth muscle cells.

- **Linalool**: Abundant in lavender, basil, and coriander, linalool possesses sedative and anxiolytic properties, which may help reduce stress-related hypertension.

Evidence-Based Benefits

Numerous studies have investigated the hypotensive effects of herbal remedies containing these plant compounds. While research is ongoing, some herbs and botanical preparations have shown promising results in clinical trials:

- **Hawthorn (Crataegus spp.)**: Rich in flavonoids and other bioactive compounds, hawthorn has been studied for its potential to lower blood pressure, improve cardiovascular function, and reduce symptoms of hypertension.

- **Garlic (Allium sativum)**: Garlic contains sulfur compounds such as allicin, which have been shown to have hypotensive effects by promoting vasodilation, inhibiting ACE, and reducing oxidative stress.

- **Hibiscus (Hibiscus sabdariffa)**: Hibiscus tea is rich in flavonoids and polyphenols, which have been associated with reductions in blood pressure in clinical studies.

Conclusion

Herbal remedies containing bioactive compounds such as flavonoids, polyphenols, alkaloids, and terpenoids offer promising options for lowering blood pressure naturally. These compounds exert their effects through various mechanisms, including vasodilation, inhibition of ACE, antioxidant activity, and modulation of endothelial function. While research on herbal remedies for hypertension continues to evolve, several herbs have demonstrated efficacy in clinical trials and are commonly used in traditional and complementary medicine practices. Incorporating these herbal remedies into a comprehensive approach to blood pressure management may offer benefits for cardiovascular health and overall well-being. However, it's important to consult with a healthcare provider before starting any herbal treatment regimen, especially if you have underlying health conditions or are taking medications, to ensure safety and effectiveness.

CHAPTER SIX

Herbal Protocol for High Blood Pressure: Dosage, Administration, and Timing

Creating a herbal protocol for high blood pressure involves careful consideration of the herbs chosen, their dosages, administration methods, and timing for optimal effectiveness. While herbal remedies can offer natural support for blood pressure management, it's crucial to develop a personalized protocol tailored to individual needs and health status. In this guide, we'll outline key factors to consider when designing a herbal protocol for high blood pressure, including dosage recommendations, administration methods, and timing considerations.

Dosage Recommendations

1. **Start Low and Go Slow**: When initiating herbal therapy for high blood pressure, it's advisable to start with lower doses and gradually increase as needed. This allows for monitoring of individual response and minimizes the risk of adverse effects.

2. **Follow Product Instructions**: Many herbal products come with recommended dosage instructions provided by the manufacturer. It's important to follow these guidelines unless otherwise directed by a qualified healthcare provider.

3. **Consult with a Herbalist or Healthcare Provider**: For personalized guidance on dosage recommendations, consult with a qualified herbalist or healthcare provider experienced in herbal medicine. They can assess your health status, consider any underlying conditions or medications, and recommend appropriate dosages tailored to your individual needs.

4. **Consider Standardized Extracts**: Some herbal supplements come in standardized extract forms, which provide consistent concentrations of active compounds. Standardized extracts can simplify dosing and ensure uniformity in potency from batch to batch.

Administration Methods

1. **Herbal Teas**: Herbal teas are a popular and traditional method of administering herbal remedies. To prepare a herbal tea, steep the desired herbs in hot water for a specified period, strain, and drink. Herbal teas can be consumed hot or cold, and their effects may vary depending on factors such as herb selection, steeping time, and frequency of consumption.

2. **Tinctures**: Tinctures are liquid extracts of herbs made by soaking plant material in alcohol or glycerin. Tinctures offer a convenient and potent way to administer herbal remedies, as they typically contain concentrated doses of active

compounds. Tinctures can be taken orally by adding drops to water or juice, and dosage can be adjusted based on individual needs.

3. **Capsules and Tablets**: Herbal supplements are available in capsule or tablet forms for convenient and standardized dosing. These dosage forms are particularly suitable for individuals who prefer a more discreet or tasteless option for herbal administration. Follow product instructions for recommended dosages and administration methods.

4. **Topical Preparations**: Some herbs can be applied topically in the form of ointments, creams, or essential oils. While topical preparations may not directly lower blood pressure, they can provide complementary benefits such as relaxation, stress reduction, and circulation support.

Timing Considerations

1. **Consistency is Key**: Establish a consistent schedule for herbal administration to maintain steady blood levels of active compounds and optimize therapeutic effects. Incorporate herbal remedies into your daily routine at consistent times to promote adherence and maximize benefits.

2. **Consider Chronobiology**: Some herbs may exhibit diurnal variations in effectiveness, meaning their effects may vary depending on the time of day. Consider timing herbal

administration based on chronobiological principles and individual response patterns.

3. **Monitor Blood Pressure**: Regularly monitor your blood pressure levels throughout the day, including before and after herbal administration. This allows for tracking of treatment efficacy and adjustment of dosages or timing as needed.

4. **Individualize Timing**: Consider individual factors such as lifestyle, meal times, medication schedules, and circadian rhythms when determining the optimal timing for herbal administration. Customize the timing of herbal remedies to fit seamlessly into your daily routine and maximize convenience and effectiveness.

Conclusion

Designing a herbal protocol for high blood pressure involves careful consideration of dosage, administration methods, and timing to optimize therapeutic outcomes. Start with low doses and gradually titrate up as needed, following product instructions or consulting with a qualified herbalist or healthcare provider for personalized guidance. Choose administration methods that align with your preferences and lifestyle, and establish a consistent schedule for herbal administration to maintain steady blood levels of active compounds. Monitor your blood pressure regularly and adjust your herbal protocol as needed based on individual response and treatment goals. With careful attention to dosage, administration, and timing, herbal remedies can be valuable components of a comprehensive approach to high blood pressure management.

CHAPTER SEVEN

Lifestyle Modifications for Blood Pressure Control: Diet, Exercise, and Stress Reduction

High blood pressure, or hypertension, is a significant risk factor for cardiovascular disease and other health complications. While medications are commonly prescribed for blood pressure management, lifestyle modifications play a crucial role in preventing and controlling hypertension. By adopting healthy habits related to diet, exercise, and stress reduction, individuals can effectively lower their blood pressure and improve overall cardiovascular health. In this guide, we'll explore evidence-based lifestyle modifications for blood pressure control, focusing on dietary strategies, exercise recommendations, and stress reduction techniques.

Dietary Strategies

1. **DASH Diet**: The Dietary Approaches to Stop Hypertension (DASH) diet is a well-established dietary pattern designed to lower blood pressure. It emphasizes consumption of fruits, vegetables, whole grains, lean proteins, and low-fat dairy products while limiting sodium, saturated fats, and added sugars. Following the DASH diet has been shown to significantly reduce blood pressure and lower the risk of cardiovascular events.

2. **Reduce Sodium Intake**: High sodium intake is strongly associated with elevated blood pressure. Limiting sodium consumption by avoiding processed foods, restaurant meals, and high-sodium condiments can help lower blood pressure levels. Aim to consume no more than 2,300 milligrams of sodium per day, or even lower if you have hypertension or are at risk for cardiovascular disease.

3. **Increase Potassium-Rich Foods**: Potassium helps regulate blood pressure by counteracting the effects of sodium and promoting vasodilation. Include potassium-rich foods such as bananas, leafy greens, sweet potatoes, avocados, and beans in your diet to support blood pressure control.

4. **Moderate Alcohol Consumption**: Excessive alcohol consumption can raise blood pressure and increase the risk of hypertension. If you choose to drink alcohol, do so in moderation, with a limit of up to one drink per day for women and up to two drinks per day for men.

5. **Limit Caffeine**: While moderate caffeine intake is generally considered safe for most individuals, excessive consumption can temporarily raise blood pressure. If you're sensitive to caffeine, consider reducing your intake or switching to decaffeinated options.

Exercise Recommendations

1. **Aerobic Exercise**: Regular aerobic exercise, such as walking, jogging, cycling, swimming, or dancing, is highly beneficial for blood pressure control. Aim for at least 150 minutes of moderate-intensity aerobic activity or 75 minutes of vigorous-intensity aerobic activity per week, spread out over several days.

2. **Strength Training**: Incorporate strength training exercises, such as weightlifting, resistance band exercises, or bodyweight exercises, into your fitness routine. Strength training helps improve muscle mass, metabolism, and cardiovascular health, contributing to lower blood pressure levels.

3. **Flexibility and Balance Exercises**: Include flexibility and balance exercises, such as yoga, tai chi, or Pilates, to enhance mobility, stability, and overall well-being. These mind-body practices can also help reduce stress and promote relaxation, further supporting blood pressure control.

4. **Consistency is Key**: Make physical activity a regular part of your daily routine by scheduling regular workouts, taking active breaks throughout the day, and incorporating enjoyable activities that keep you moving and motivated.

Stress Reduction Techniques

1. **Mindfulness Meditation**: Practice mindfulness meditation to cultivate present-moment awareness and reduce stress levels. Mindfulness techniques, such as deep breathing, body scanning, and guided imagery, can help promote relaxation and lower blood pressure.

2. **Progressive Muscle Relaxation**: Engage in progressive muscle relaxation exercises to release tension and promote physical and mental relaxation. This technique involves systematically tensing and relaxing muscle groups throughout the body, helping to alleviate stress and reduce blood pressure.

3. **Yoga and Tai Chi**: Participate in yoga or tai chi classes to improve flexibility, balance, and mental well-being. These mind-body practices combine physical postures, breathing techniques, and meditation to promote relaxation and stress reduction, which can contribute to lower blood pressure levels over time.

4. **Healthy Coping Mechanisms**: Identify healthy coping mechanisms for managing stress, such as spending time in nature, engaging in creative activities, connecting with loved ones, or seeking support from a therapist or counselor. Avoid using unhealthy coping strategies such as smoking,

excessive alcohol consumption, or overeating, which can worsen blood pressure and overall health.

Conclusion

Incorporating lifestyle modifications related to diet, exercise, and stress reduction is essential for blood pressure control and overall cardiovascular health. By adopting a DASH-style diet rich in fruits, vegetables, and whole grains, reducing sodium intake, and limiting alcohol and caffeine consumption, individuals can support healthy blood pressure levels. Regular physical activity, including aerobic exercise, strength training, and mind-body practices, helps improve cardiovascular fitness, reduce stress, and lower blood pressure. Additionally, incorporating stress reduction techniques such as mindfulness meditation, progressive muscle relaxation, and yoga can promote relaxation and well-being. By implementing these evidence-based lifestyle modifications, individuals can take proactive steps toward preventing and managing hypertension, ultimately reducing their risk of cardiovascular disease and improving long-term health outcomes.

CHAPTER EIGHT

Monitoring Blood Pressure: How to Track Progress and Adjust Treatment

Monitoring blood pressure regularly is essential for effectively managing hypertension and evaluating the effectiveness of treatment strategies. By tracking blood pressure readings over time and making adjustments based on trends and individual response, individuals can optimize their treatment approach and reduce the risk of cardiovascular complications. In this guide, we'll explore strategies for monitoring blood pressure, including frequency of measurements, interpreting readings, and adjusting treatment as needed to achieve optimal blood pressure control.

Frequency of Blood Pressure Measurements

1. **Regular Monitoring**: Individuals with hypertension or those at risk for high blood pressure should monitor their blood pressure regularly, as advised by their healthcare provider. Frequency of measurements may vary depending on factors such as baseline blood pressure levels, treatment goals, and overall health status.

2. **Home Blood Pressure Monitoring**: Home blood pressure monitoring is a valuable tool for tracking blood pressure outside of clinical settings and provides a more comprehensive picture of daily fluctuations. It allows

individuals to monitor their blood pressure at different times of the day and in various situations, such as before and after meals, exercise, or stressors.

3. **Recommended Schedule**: The American Heart Association (AHA) recommends monitoring blood pressure at least twice daily, preferably in the morning and evening, using a validated home blood pressure monitor. Keep a log of blood pressure readings, including date, time, and any relevant factors such as medication doses, physical activity, or dietary changes.

Interpreting Blood Pressure Readings

1. **Understanding Blood Pressure Numbers**: Blood pressure readings consist of two numbers: systolic pressure (the top number) and diastolic pressure (the bottom number), measured in millimeters of mercury (mm Hg). Normal blood pressure is typically defined as less than 120/80 mm Hg, while hypertension is diagnosed when blood pressure consistently exceeds 130/80 mm Hg.

2. **Target Blood Pressure Goals**: Treatment goals for blood pressure management may vary depending on individual risk factors and health conditions. For most individuals with hypertension, the target blood pressure goal is less than 130/80 mm Hg. However, certain populations, such as older

adults or those with underlying health conditions, may have different target goals.

3. **Recognizing Patterns and Trends**: Pay attention to patterns and trends in blood pressure readings over time. Look for consistent patterns of elevated blood pressure, fluctuations throughout the day, or changes in response to treatment interventions. Identify any factors or triggers that may influence blood pressure levels, such as stress, medication adherence, or lifestyle habits.

Adjusting Treatment Based on Blood Pressure Trends

1. **Consult with a Healthcare Provider**: Discuss blood pressure trends and treatment adjustments with a qualified healthcare provider, such as a primary care physician, cardiologist, or hypertension specialist. Share your home blood pressure log and any observations or concerns regarding treatment efficacy or side effects.

2. **Medication Adjustments**: If blood pressure remains elevated despite lifestyle modifications and initial medication therapy, healthcare providers may consider adjusting medication doses, adding or switching to alternative medications, or combining multiple antihypertensive agents to achieve optimal blood pressure control.

3. **Lifestyle Modifications**: Reinforce the importance of lifestyle modifications for blood pressure management, including dietary changes, regular exercise, stress reduction techniques, and medication adherence. Encourage individuals to make sustainable lifestyle changes and provide support and resources to help them achieve their goals.

4. **Regular Follow-Up**: Schedule regular follow-up appointments with healthcare providers to assess treatment response, monitor blood pressure trends, and adjust treatment as needed. Periodic reassessment allows for ongoing optimization of treatment strategies and evaluation of long-term cardiovascular risk reduction.

Conclusion

Monitoring blood pressure regularly and making adjustments to treatment based on trends and individual response are essential components of hypertension management. By tracking blood pressure readings at home and maintaining a log of measurements, individuals can gain valuable insights into their blood pressure patterns and treatment efficacy. Interpretation of blood pressure readings involves understanding target goals, recognizing patterns and trends, and identifying factors that may influence blood pressure levels. Healthcare providers play a crucial role in guiding treatment adjustments, including medication optimization, lifestyle modifications, and ongoing monitoring of cardiovascular risk factors. By working collaboratively with healthcare providers and actively participating in blood pressure management, individuals can achieve optimal blood pressure control and reduce their risk of cardiovascular complications.

CHAPTER NINE

Integrating Herbal Remedies with Conventional Treatment: Benefits and Considerations

Integrating herbal remedies with conventional treatment offers a holistic approach to healthcare, combining the best of both traditional and modern medicine to optimize patient outcomes. While conventional treatments such as medications are often the first line of defense for many health conditions, herbal remedies can complement these therapies by addressing underlying imbalances, minimizing side effects, and promoting overall well-being. In this guide, we'll explore the benefits and considerations of integrating herbal remedies with conventional treatment, providing insights into how this approach can enhance patient care and improve health outcomes.

Benefits of Integrating Herbal Remedies with Conventional Treatment

1. **Comprehensive Approach to Healing**: Herbal remedies offer a holistic approach to health and wellness, addressing not only symptoms but also underlying imbalances and contributing factors. By targeting multiple aspects of health, herbal remedies complement conventional treatments and promote comprehensive healing.

2. **Reduced Side Effects**: Herbal remedies often have fewer side effects compared to conventional medications, making them attractive options for individuals who experience adverse reactions or intolerances to pharmaceutical drugs. Integrating herbal remedies with conventional treatment can help minimize side effects and enhance treatment tolerability.

3. **Support for Long-Term Management**: Herbal remedies can play a valuable role in long-term disease management by providing ongoing support for health and well-being. Unlike some pharmaceutical drugs that may be used for short-term symptom relief, herbal remedies can be incorporated into daily routines to maintain balance and prevent disease recurrence.

4. **Individualized Treatment Options**: Herbal medicine offers a wide range of remedies that can be tailored to individual needs and preferences. Herbalists and healthcare providers can personalize treatment plans based on factors such as patient history, constitution, lifestyle, and treatment goals, ensuring that each individual receives personalized care.

5. **Promotion of Self-Care and Empowerment**: Integrating herbal remedies empowers individuals to take an active role in their health and well-being. By learning about herbal medicine, making informed choices, and actively

participating in treatment decisions, individuals become more engaged in their own care and gain a sense of empowerment over their health.

Considerations for Integrating Herbal Remedies with Conventional Treatment

1. **Safety and Efficacy**: While many herbal remedies have a long history of traditional use and anecdotal evidence supporting their efficacy, not all herbal products have been rigorously studied in clinical trials. It's essential to choose high-quality herbal products from reputable sources and consult with qualified healthcare providers to ensure safety and efficacy.

2. **Potential Interactions with Medications**: Herbal remedies have the potential to interact with conventional medications, altering their efficacy or increasing the risk of adverse effects. Healthcare providers should carefully evaluate potential herb-drug interactions and consider factors such as dosage, timing, and patient health status when integrating herbal remedies with conventional treatment.

3. **Patient Education and Informed Consent**: Patients should be educated about the risks and benefits of integrating herbal remedies with conventional treatment and provide informed consent before starting herbal therapy. Healthcare providers play a crucial role in educating patients about herbal

medicine, addressing any concerns or misconceptions, and facilitating shared decision-making.

4. **Monitoring and Follow-Up**: Regular monitoring and follow-up are essential when integrating herbal remedies with conventional treatment. Healthcare providers should track patient progress, monitor for potential adverse effects or interactions, and adjust treatment plans as needed to optimize outcomes.

5. **Integration with Conventional Care**: Herbal remedies should complement, not replace, conventional treatments prescribed by healthcare providers. It's important to integrate herbal therapy into existing treatment plans in a coordinated and collaborative manner, ensuring seamless communication and coordination of care between herbalists and conventional healthcare providers.

Conclusion

Integrating herbal remedies with conventional treatment offers numerous benefits for patient care, including a comprehensive approach to healing, reduced side effects, long-term support for health management, individualized treatment options, and promotion of self-care and empowerment. However, it's essential to consider safety, potential interactions with medications, patient education and informed consent, monitoring and follow-up, and integration with conventional care when incorporating herbal therapy into treatment plans. By navigating these considerations thoughtfully and collaboratively, healthcare providers can harness the synergistic potential of herbal remedies and conventional treatments to optimize patient outcomes and promote holistic health and well-being.

CHAPTER TEN

Long-Term Maintenance: Sustaining Healthy Blood Pressure Levels with Herbal Support

Maintaining healthy blood pressure levels over the long term is essential for preventing cardiovascular disease and promoting overall well-being. While lifestyle modifications and conventional medications play crucial roles in blood pressure management, herbal support can complement these approaches by providing ongoing support for cardiovascular health. In this guide, we'll explore strategies for sustaining healthy blood pressure levels with herbal support, including herbal remedies, lifestyle modifications, and considerations for long-term maintenance.

Herbal Remedies for Long-Term Blood Pressure Maintenance

1. **Hawthorn (Crataegus spp.)**: Hawthorn is a well-known herb with cardiovascular benefits, including its ability to support healthy blood pressure levels. It contains flavonoids and other bioactive compounds that promote blood vessel health, improve circulation, and regulate blood pressure. Hawthorn can be consumed as a tea, tincture, or standardized extract for long-term maintenance of cardiovascular health.

2. **Garlic (Allium sativum)**: Garlic has been used for centuries for its medicinal properties, including its potential to lower

blood pressure. Allicin, a sulfur-containing compound found in garlic, has vasodilatory effects and may help reduce blood pressure levels over time. Incorporating fresh garlic into cooking or taking garlic supplements can provide long-term cardiovascular support.

3. **Olive Leaf (Olea europaea)**: Olive leaf extract contains oleuropein and other phenolic compounds with antioxidant and anti-inflammatory properties, which may contribute to its ability to support healthy blood pressure levels. Olive leaf extract can be taken as a supplement for long-term cardiovascular maintenance.

4. **Hibiscus (Hibiscus sabdariffa)**: Hibiscus tea is rich in flavonoids and polyphenols that have been shown to have hypotensive effects. Drinking hibiscus tea regularly may help maintain healthy blood pressure levels over time. Enjoying a cup of hibiscus tea as part of a daily routine can provide ongoing cardiovascular support.

5. **Astragalus (Astragalus membranaceus)**: Astragalus is an herb used in traditional Chinese medicine for its cardiovascular benefits, including its potential to support healthy blood pressure levels. Astragalus may help improve endothelial function, reduce oxidative stress, and promote overall cardiovascular health. Incorporating astragalus into

herbal formulations or taking it as a supplement can provide long-term cardiovascular support.

Lifestyle Modifications for Long-Term Blood Pressure Maintenance

1. **Healthy Diet**: Adopting a balanced diet rich in fruits, vegetables, whole grains, lean proteins, and healthy fats can support long-term blood pressure maintenance. Limiting sodium, saturated fats, and added sugars while increasing potassium-rich foods can help promote cardiovascular health.

2. **Regular Exercise**: Engaging in regular physical activity, including aerobic exercise, strength training, and flexibility exercises, can support long-term blood pressure control. Aim for at least 150 minutes of moderate-intensity aerobic activity or 75 minutes of vigorous-intensity aerobic activity per week, along with muscle-strengthening activities on two or more days per week.

3. **Stress Management**: Chronic stress can contribute to elevated blood pressure levels over time. Incorporating stress-reducing practices such as mindfulness meditation, deep breathing exercises, yoga, or tai chi into daily routines can help promote relaxation and support long-term cardiovascular health.

4. **Maintaining a Healthy Weight**: Achieving and maintaining a healthy weight is important for blood pressure management. Losing excess weight through a combination of diet and exercise can help reduce blood pressure levels and support long-term cardiovascular health.

5. **Regular Monitoring and Follow-Up**: Regular monitoring of blood pressure levels and periodic follow-up with healthcare providers are essential for long-term blood pressure maintenance. Healthcare providers can assess treatment effectiveness, monitor for any changes in blood pressure, and make adjustments to treatment plans as needed to optimize cardiovascular health.

Considerations for Long-Term Maintenance

1. **Consistency is Key**: Consistency in herbal supplementation, dietary habits, exercise routines, and stress management practices is crucial for long-term blood pressure maintenance. Establishing healthy habits and incorporating them into daily routines can support ongoing cardiovascular health.

2. **Individualized Approach**: Blood pressure management should be tailored to individual needs, preferences, and health status. Working with a qualified healthcare provider or herbalist can help develop a personalized treatment plan

that addresses specific concerns and optimizes long-term cardiovascular health.

3. **Adherence to Treatment Plan**: Adherence to the treatment plan, including herbal supplementation, lifestyle modifications, and prescribed medications, is essential for long-term blood pressure maintenance. Patients should communicate openly with healthcare providers about any challenges or concerns regarding treatment adherence and seek support as needed.

4. **Regular Evaluation and Adjustment**: Regular evaluation of blood pressure levels and treatment effectiveness is necessary for long-term maintenance. Healthcare providers can monitor progress, assess any changes in health status, and make adjustments to treatment plans as needed to achieve optimal cardiovascular health outcomes.

Conclusion

Sustaining healthy blood pressure levels over the long term requires a comprehensive approach that integrates herbal support with lifestyle modifications and regular monitoring. Herbal remedies such as hawthorn, garlic, olive leaf, hibiscus, and astragalus can provide ongoing cardiovascular support and complement lifestyle modifications aimed at maintaining healthy blood pressure levels. By adopting a balanced diet, engaging in regular physical activity, managing stress effectively, and adhering to treatment plans, individuals can support long-term blood pressure maintenance and reduce their risk of cardiovascular disease. Working collaboratively with healthcare providers and herbalists can help develop personalized treatment plans that address individual needs and optimize cardiovascular health outcomes over time.

BONUS: SOME VITAL HERBAL REMEDIES FOR HEALTH AND WELLNESS

Bladderwrack:

Definition: Bladderwrack is a type of seaweed or marine algae commonly used in traditional medicine and as a dietary supplement. It's known for its potential health benefits, particularly related to thyroid health and weight management.

Ingredients: Bladderwrack contains various nutrients, including iodine, vitamins, minerals, and antioxidants. The primary active components are iodine and fucoidan, a type of carbohydrate found in brown seaweeds.

How to Prepare: Bladderwrack supplements are available in various forms, including capsules, powders, and liquid extracts. They can be taken orally with water or added to smoothies and other beverages.

Dosage: The appropriate dosage of bladderwrack can vary based on factors such as age, health status, and the specific product being used. It's essential to follow the recommended dosage on the product label or consult with a healthcare professional for personalized guidance.

How to Use: Bladderwrack supplements are typically taken orally, either with water or mixed into food or beverages. It's important to follow the instructions on the product label and avoid exceeding the recommended dosage.

Side Effects: While bladderwrack is generally considered safe for most people when used in moderation, excessive intake of iodine from bladderwrack supplements can cause thyroid dysfunction and other adverse effects. Individuals with thyroid disorders, iodine sensitivity, or certain medical conditions should exercise caution and consult with a healthcare provider before using bladderwrack supplements. Common side effects may include digestive upset, allergic reactions, or interactions with medications.

Blood Purifier:

Definition: Blood purifiers are herbal remedies or dietary supplements believed to cleanse or detoxify the blood, often promoting overall health and well-being. They are thought to support the body's natural detoxification processes and improve blood circulation.

Ingredients: Blood purifiers may contain a variety of herbs and botanical extracts known for their purported cleansing and detoxifying properties. Common ingredients include burdock root, red clover, dandelion root, and yellow dock root, among others.

How to Prepare: Blood purifiers are typically available in various forms, including capsules, tablets, powders, and liquid extracts. They are usually taken orally with water or juice, following the recommended dosage on the product label.

Dosage: The dosage of blood purifiers can vary depending on the specific product and individual needs. It's important to adhere to the recommended dosage on the product label or consult with a healthcare professional for personalized guidance.

How to Use: Blood purifiers are typically taken orally, either with water or mixed into beverages. They are often used as part of a detoxification regimen or to support overall health and vitality.

Side Effects: While blood purifiers are generally considered safe for most people when used as directed, some individuals may experience side effects such as digestive discomfort, allergic reactions, or interactions with medications. It's important to consult with a healthcare provider before starting any new supplement regimen, especially if you have underlying health conditions or are taking medications.

Blue Vervain:

Definition: Blue vervain, also known as Verbena hastata, is a perennial herb native to North America. It has been used in traditional medicine for centuries to treat various ailments, including anxiety, insomnia, and digestive issues.

Ingredients: Blue vervain contains several active compounds, including aucubin, verbenalin, and volatile oils. These compounds are believed to contribute to the herb's medicinal properties.

How to Prepare: Blue vervain is typically consumed as a tea or tincture. To make tea, dried blue vervain leaves and flowers are steeped in hot water for several minutes before being strained and consumed. Tinctures are prepared by steeping the herb in alcohol or vinegar to extract its active compounds.

Dosage: The appropriate dosage of blue vervain can vary depending on factors such as age, health status, and the specific preparation being used. It's important to follow the recommended dosage on the product label or consult with a qualified herbalist or healthcare professional for personalized guidance.

How to Use: Blue vervain tea or tincture is typically taken orally. It can be consumed on its own or mixed with honey or other herbal teas for added flavor.

Side Effects: While blue vervain is generally considered safe for most people when used in moderation, excessive intake may cause digestive upset or allergic reactions in some individuals. Pregnant or breastfeeding women should avoid blue vervain due to its potential to stimulate uterine contractions. As with any herbal remedy, it's important to consult with a healthcare provider before using blue vervain, especially if you have underlying health conditions or are taking medications.

Burdock:

Definition: Burdock, scientifically known as Arctium lappa, is a biennial plant native to Europe and Asia but now found worldwide. It's part of the Asteraceae family and has been used for centuries in traditional medicine and culinary practices.

Ingredients: Burdock contains various nutrients, including carbohydrates, fiber, vitamins (such as vitamin B6, folate, and vitamin C), and minerals (including potassium, magnesium, and manganese). It also contains active compounds such as polyphenols and volatile oils.

How to Prepare: Burdock can be prepared and consumed in various ways. The roots, leaves, and seeds are all utilized for different purposes. The root is commonly used in cooking, herbal teas, tinctures, and supplements, while the leaves and seeds are sometimes used in herbal preparations.

Dosage: The appropriate dosage of burdock root can vary depending on the specific form and intended use. For culinary purposes, there are no strict dosage guidelines, but for supplements or herbal remedies, it's essential to follow the recommended dosage on the product label or consult with a healthcare professional.

How to Use: Burdock root can be used in cooking by peeling, slicing, and adding it to soups, stews, stir-fries, or salads. It can also be brewed into a tea or used to make tinctures or extracts for medicinal purposes. Some people may also take burdock root supplements in capsule or powder form.

Side Effects: While burdock is generally considered safe for most people when consumed in moderate amounts, some individuals may experience allergic reactions or digestive upset. Additionally, burdock may interact with certain medications or have adverse effects in individuals with certain health conditions, such as diabetes or allergies to plants in the Asteraceae family. It's important to consult with a healthcare provider before using burdock, especially if you have underlying health conditions or are taking medications.

Cascara Sagrada:

Definition: Cascara Sagrada, scientifically known as Rhamnus purshiana, is a species of buckthorn native to western North America. It has been used traditionally as a laxative and to promote bowel regularity.

Ingredients: The primary active ingredients in cascara sagrada are anthraquinone glycosides, particularly cascarosides A and B. These compounds stimulate peristalsis in the colon, leading to increased bowel movements.

How to Prepare: Cascara sagrada is typically prepared as an herbal tea, tincture, or capsule. To make tea, dried cascara sagrada bark is steeped in hot water for several minutes before being strained and consumed. Tinctures are prepared by steeping the bark in alcohol to extract its active compounds.

Dosage: The appropriate dosage of cascara sagrada can vary depending on the specific preparation and intended use. It's important to follow the recommended dosage on the product label or consult with a healthcare professional for personalized guidance.

How to Use: Cascara sagrada tea or tincture is typically taken orally. It's important to start with a low dose and gradually increase if needed to avoid potential side effects such as cramping or diarrhea.

Side Effects: Cascara sagrada is considered safe for short-term use when used as directed. However, long-term or excessive use may lead to dependence, electrolyte imbalance, or dehydration. It may also interact with certain medications or have adverse effects in individuals with certain health conditions. It's important to use cascara sagrada under the guidance of a healthcare professional and to discontinue use if any adverse effects occur.

Cell Food:

Definition: Cell Food is a dietary supplement marketed as a highly oxygenating and alkalizing formula. It's claimed to support overall health and vitality by providing essential nutrients and oxygen to the cells.

Ingredients: The exact ingredients of Cell Food can vary depending on the brand, but it typically contains a proprietary blend of minerals, enzymes, electrolytes, and trace elements. Some common ingredients may include purified water, dissolved oxygen, seawater extract, and plant-based enzymes.

How to Prepare: Cell Food is usually available in liquid form and is typically taken orally. It can be consumed directly or diluted in water or juice before consumption.

Dosage: The dosage of Cell Food can vary depending on the specific product and individual needs. It's important to follow the recommended dosage on the product label or consult with a healthcare professional for personalized guidance.

How to Use: Cell Food is typically taken orally, either directly or mixed into water or juice. It's important to shake the bottle well before use and to store it according to the manufacturer's instructions.

Side Effects: Cell Food is generally considered safe for most people when used as directed. However, some individuals may experience mild digestive upset or allergic reactions to certain ingredients. It's essential to consult with a healthcare provider before starting any new supplement regimen, especially if you have underlying health conditions or are taking medications.

Chaparral:

Definition: Chaparral, scientifically known as Larrea tridentata, is a shrub native to the southwestern United States and northern Mexico. It has been used for centuries by Native American tribes for its medicinal properties and is commonly used in herbal medicine today.

Ingredients: Chaparral contains several bioactive compounds, including nordihydroguaiaretic acid (NDGA), flavonoids, lignans, and volatile oils. NDGA is believed to be the primary active compound responsible for many of chaparral's therapeutic effects.

How to Prepare: Chaparral can be prepared and consumed in various forms, including teas, tinctures, capsules, and topical preparations. To make tea, dried chaparral leaves are steeped in hot water for several minutes before being strained and consumed. Tinctures are prepared by steeping the herb in alcohol or vinegar to extract its active compounds.

Dosage: The appropriate dosage of chaparral can vary depending on the specific form and intended use. It's important to follow the recommended dosage on the product label or consult with a healthcare professional for personalized guidance.

How to Use: Chaparral tea or tincture is typically taken orally. It can also be applied topically to the skin for certain conditions. It's important to use chaparral products as directed and to discontinue use if any adverse effects occur.

Side Effects: Chaparral is generally considered safe for most people when used in moderate amounts. However, excessive intake or prolonged use may lead to liver toxicity or other adverse effects. It may also interact with certain medications or have adverse effects in individuals with certain health conditions. It's important to use chaparral under the guidance of a healthcare professional and to discontinue use if any adverse effects occur.

Cocolmeca:

Definition: Cocolmeca, also known as Smilax ornata or sarsaparilla, is a flowering vine native to Mexico and Central America. It has been used traditionally in Mexican and Central American folk medicine for its purported medicinal properties.

Ingredients: Cocolmeca contains various bioactive compounds, including saponins, flavonoids, and plant sterols. These compounds are believed to contribute to the herb's medicinal properties, including its potential as a diuretic, blood purifier, and anti-inflammatory agent.

How to Prepare: Cocolmeca is commonly prepared and consumed as an herbal tea or decoction. To make tea, dried cocolmeca roots or leaves are steeped in hot water for several minutes before being strained and consumed. Decoctions involve boiling the roots or leaves in water to extract their active compounds.

Dosage: The appropriate dosage of cocolmeca can vary depending on factors such as age, health status, and the specific preparation being used. It's important to follow the recommended dosage on the product label or consult with a qualified herbalist or healthcare professional for personalized guidance.

How to Use: Cocolmeca tea or decoction is typically taken orally. It can also be used topically for certain skin conditions. It's important to use cocolmeca products as directed and to discontinue use if any adverse effects occur.

Side Effects: Cocolmeca is generally considered safe for most people when used in moderate amounts. However, excessive intake may lead to digestive upset or other adverse effects. It may also interact with certain medications or have adverse effects in individuals with certain health conditions. It's important to use cocolmeca under the guidance of a healthcare professional and to discontinue use if any adverse effects occur.

Contribo:

Definition: Contribo, also known as Aristolochiatrilobata, is a vine native to the Caribbean and Central America. It has been used traditionally in folk medicine for various purposes, including as a remedy for digestive issues, inflammation, and pain relief.

Ingredients: Contribo contains several bioactive compounds, including aristolochic acids, flavonoids, and alkaloids. These compounds are believed to contribute to the herb's medicinal properties, including its potential as an anti-inflammatory and analgesic agent.

How to Prepare: Contribo is typically prepared and consumed as an herbal tea or decoction. To make tea, dried contribo leaves or stems are steeped in hot water for several minutes before being strained and consumed. Decoctions involve boiling the leaves or stems in water to extract their active compounds.

Dosage: The appropriate dosage of contribo can vary depending on factors such as age, health status, and the specific preparation being used. It's important to follow the recommended dosage on the product label or consult with a qualified herbalist or healthcare professional for personalized guidance.

How to Use: Contribo tea or decoction is typically taken orally. It's important to use contribo products as directed and to discontinue use if any adverse effects occur.

Side Effects: Contribo contains aristolochic acids, which have been associated with serious adverse effects, including kidney damage and cancer. Due to these safety concerns, the use of contribo is highly discouraged, and it's important to avoid products containing aristolochic acids. Individuals should seek alternative remedies for their health needs.

Herban Iron:

Definition: Herban Iron is a dietary supplement designed to provide an easily absorbable form of iron to support healthy iron levels in the body. It's particularly beneficial for individuals with iron deficiency or anemia.

Ingredients: Herban Iron typically contains iron in the form of ferrous bisglycinate, which is a highly bioavailable and gentle form of iron that is less likely to cause digestive upset or constipation compared to other forms of iron. It may also contain other ingredients such as vitamin C to enhance iron absorption.

How to Prepare: Herban Iron is usually available in capsule or liquid form. Capsules are taken orally with water, while liquid forms may be mixed with water or juice before consumption. It's important to follow the recommended dosage on the product label.

Dosage: The appropriate dosage of Herban Iron depends on factors such as age, gender, and the severity of iron deficiency.

It's important to consult with a healthcare professional to determine the correct dosage for individual needs.

How to Use: Herban Iron capsules are typically taken orally with water, while liquid forms may be mixed with water or juice before consumption. It's important to take Herban Iron as directed and to avoid taking it with dairy products, antacids, or other substances that may interfere with iron absorption.

Side Effects: While Herban Iron is generally considered safe for most people when used as directed, some individuals may experience mild side effects such as gastrointestinal discomfort or constipation. It's important to consult with a healthcare professional before starting any new supplement regimen, especially if you have underlying health conditions or are taking medications.

Hydrangea:

Definition: Hydrangea, scientifically known as Hydrangea arborescens, is a flowering shrub native to North America. It has been used traditionally in herbal medicine for its potential diuretic and anti-inflammatory properties.

Ingredients: Hydrangea contains several bioactive compounds, including saponins, flavonoids, and glycosides. These compounds are believed to contribute to the herb's medicinal properties, including its potential as a diuretic, kidney tonic, and anti-inflammatory agent.

How to Prepare: Hydrangea root is typically prepared and consumed as an herbal tea or tincture. To make tea, dried hydrangea root is steeped in hot water for several minutes before being strained and consumed. Tinctures are prepared by steeping the root in alcohol or vinegar to extract its active compounds.

Dosage: The appropriate dosage of hydrangea can vary depending on factors such as age, health status, and the specific preparation being used. It's important to follow the recommended dosage on the product label or consult with a qualified herbalist or healthcare professional for personalized guidance.

How to Use: Hydrangea tea or tincture is typically taken orally. It's important to use hydrangea products as directed and to discontinue use if any adverse effects occur.

Side Effects: Hydrangea is generally considered safe for most people when used in moderate amounts. However, some individuals may experience digestive upset or allergic reactions. It may also interact with certain medications or have adverse effects in individuals with certain health conditions. It's important to use hydrangea under the guidance of a healthcare professional and to discontinue use if any adverse effects occur.

Manjakani:

Definition: Manjakani, also known as Quercus infectoria or oak gall, is a natural substance derived from the oak tree. It has been used for centuries in traditional medicine for its potential health benefits, particularly for women's health and vaginal tightening.

Ingredients: Manjakani contains various bioactive compounds, including tannins, flavonoids, and gallic acid. These compounds are believed to contribute to the herb's medicinal properties, including its potential as an astringent and antiseptic agent.

How to Prepare: Manjakani is typically available in powder, capsule, or liquid extract form. It can be taken orally or used topically depending on the intended use. For vaginal tightening, manjakani may be applied topically as a gel or inserted into the vagina in capsule form.

Dosage: The appropriate dosage of manjakani can vary depending on factors such as age, health status, and the specific preparation being used. It's important to follow the recommended dosage on the product label or consult with a qualified herbalist or healthcare professional for personalized guidance.

How to Use: Manjakani can be taken orally or used topically depending on the intended use. It's important to use manjakani products as directed and to discontinue use if any adverse effects occur.

Side Effects: Manjakani is generally considered safe for most people when used in moderate amounts. However, some individuals may experience allergic reactions or skin irritation when used topically. It's important to use manjakani under the guidance of a healthcare professional and to discontinue use if any adverse effects occur.

Irish Moss:

Definition: Irish Moss, scientifically known as Chondrus crispus, is a species of red algae or seaweed native to the Atlantic coastlines of Europe and North America. It has been used for centuries in traditional Irish and Scottish cuisine, as well as in herbal medicine.

Ingredients: Irish Moss is rich in various nutrients, including iodine, sulfur compounds, vitamins (such as vitamin A, vitamin K, and vitamin B12), minerals (including calcium, magnesium, potassium, and sodium), and polysaccharides (such as carrageenan). These nutrients are believed to contribute to the herb's potential health benefits.

How to Prepare: Irish Moss is typically prepared by soaking it in water to rehydrate and soften it before use. It can be added to soups, stews, smoothies, desserts, and other dishes as a thickening agent or nutritional supplement.

Dosage: The appropriate dosage of Irish Moss can vary depending on factors such as age, health status, and the specific preparation being used. It's important to follow recipes or guidelines for culinary use and to consult with a healthcare professional for guidance on using Irish Moss as a dietary supplement.

How to Use: Irish Moss can be used in culinary applications to add thickness and nutritional value to dishes. It can also be consumed as a dietary supplement in the form of capsules, powders, or extracts.

Side Effects: Irish Moss is generally considered safe for most people when consumed in moderate amounts as part of a balanced diet. However, some individuals may be allergic to seaweed or carrageenan, a compound found in Irish Moss that is used as a food additive. It's important to discontinue use if any adverse effects occur and to consult with a healthcare professional if you have any concerns.

Irish Sea Moss:

Definition: Irish Sea Moss is a term often used interchangeably with Irish Moss, referring to the same species of red algae, Chondrus crispus. It's harvested from the rocky shores of the Atlantic coastlines of Europe and North America.

Ingredients: Irish Sea Moss shares the same nutritional profile as Irish Moss, containing iodine, vitamins, minerals, and polysaccharides. It's valued for its potential health benefits, including supporting thyroid function, boosting immune health, and promoting digestion.

How to Prepare: Irish Sea Moss is prepared in the same way as Irish Moss, by soaking it in water to rehydrate and soften it before use. It can be used in culinary applications or consumed as a dietary supplement.

Dosage: The dosage of Irish Sea Moss depends on the form and intended use. As a dietary supplement, it's important to follow the recommended dosage on the product label or consult with a healthcare professional for personalized guidance.

How to Use: Irish Sea Moss can be used in various culinary applications, including soups, smoothies, desserts, and sauces. It can also be consumed as a dietary supplement in the form of capsules, powders, or extracts.

Side Effects: Similar to Irish Moss, Irish Sea Moss is generally considered safe for most people when consumed in moderate amounts. However, individuals with seaweed allergies or sensitivities to carrageenan should exercise caution. It's important to discontinue use if any adverse effects occur and to consult with a healthcare professional if you have any concerns.

Lymphalin:

Definition: Lymphalin is a herbal supplement formulated to support lymphatic system health. The lymphatic system plays a crucial role in immune function and waste removal in the body, and Lymphalin is designed to promote its proper function.

Ingredients: Lymphalin typically contains a blend of herbs and botanical extracts known for their traditional use in supporting lymphatic system health. Common ingredients may include cleavers, red clover, echinacea, burdock root, and calendula, among others.

How to Prepare: Lymphalin is usually available in capsule or liquid form. Capsules are taken orally with water, while liquid forms may be mixed with water or juice before consumption. It's important to follow the recommended dosage on the product label.

Dosage: The appropriate dosage of Lymphalin can vary depending on the specific product and individual needs. It's important to follow the recommended dosage on the product label or consult with a healthcare professional for personalized guidance.

How to Use: Lymphalin capsules are typically taken orally with water, while liquid forms may be mixed with water or juice before consumption. It's often recommended to take Lymphalin on an empty stomach for optimal absorption.

Side Effects: Lymphalin is generally considered safe for most people when used as directed. However, some individuals may experience mild side effects such as gastrointestinal discomfort or allergic reactions to certain ingredients. It's important to consult with a healthcare provider before starting any new supplement regimen, especially if you have underlying health conditions or are taking medications.

Dandelion Root:

Definition: Dandelion, scientifically known as Taraxacum officinale, is a common flowering plant found worldwide. While often considered a pesky weed, dandelion has a long history of use in traditional medicine for its various health benefits.

Ingredients: Dandelion root contains several bioactive compounds, including sesquiterpene lactones, triterpenes, flavonoids, and polysaccharides. These compounds are believed to contribute to the herb's medicinal properties, including its potential as a diuretic, digestive aid, and liver tonic.

How to Prepare: Dandelion root can be prepared and consumed in various forms, including teas, tinctures, capsules, and extracts. To make tea, dried dandelion root is steeped in hot water for several minutes before being strained and consumed. Tinctures are prepared by steeping the root in alcohol or vinegar to extract its active compounds.

Dosage: The appropriate dosage of dandelion root can vary depending on factors such as age, health status, and the specific preparation being used. It's important to follow the recommended dosage on the product label or consult with a qualified herbalist or healthcare professional for personalized guidance.

How to Use: Dandelion root tea, tincture, or capsules are typically taken orally. It's important to use dandelion root products as directed and to discontinue use if any adverse effects occur.

Side Effects: Dandelion root is generally considered safe for most people when used in moderate amounts. However, some individuals may experience allergic reactions or digestive upset. It may also interact with certain medications or have adverse effects in individuals with certain health conditions. It's important to use dandelion root under the guidance of a healthcare professional and to discontinue use if any adverse effects occur.

Green Food Plus:

Definition: Green Food Plus is a dietary supplement formulated to provide a concentrated source of nutrients derived from various green plants. It's designed to support overall health and well-being by delivering essential vitamins, minerals, antioxidants, and phytonutrients.

Ingredients: Green Food Plus typically contains a blend of powdered green vegetables, grasses, algae, and other plant-based ingredients. Common ingredients may include wheatgrass, barley grass, spirulina, chlorella, alfalfa, kale, spinach, and broccoli, among others.

How to Prepare: Green Food Plus is usually available in powder form and can be mixed with water, juice, or smoothies. It's important to follow the recommended dosage on the product label and to consume it as part of a balanced diet.

Dosage: The appropriate dosage of Green Food Plus can vary depending on the specific product and individual needs. It's important to follow the recommended dosage on the product label or consult with a healthcare professional for personalized guidance.

How to Use: Green Food Plus powder is typically mixed with water, juice, or smoothies and consumed orally. It's often taken once or twice daily, preferably with meals, to maximize nutrient absorption.

Side Effects: Green Food Plus is generally considered safe for most people when used as directed. However, some individuals may experience digestive upset or allergic reactions to certain ingredients. It's important to consult with a healthcare provider before starting any new supplement regimen, especially if you have underlying health conditions or are taking medications.

Guaco:

Definition: Guaco, also known as Mikania cordata or Mikania glomerata, is a medicinal plant native to Central and South America. It has a long history of use in traditional medicine for its potential therapeutic properties.

Ingredients: Guaco contains several bioactive compounds, including coumarins, flavonoids, tannins, and saponins. These compounds are believed to contribute to the herb's medicinal properties, including its potential as an expectorant, anti-inflammatory, and antispasmodic agent.

How to Prepare: Guaco is typically prepared and consumed as an herbal tea or infusion. To make tea, dried guaco leaves are steeped in hot water for several minutes before being strained and consumed.

Dosage: The appropriate dosage of guaco can vary depending on factors such as age, health status, and the specific preparation being used. It's important to follow the recommended dosage on the product label or consult with a qualified herbalist or healthcare professional for personalized guidance.

How to Use: Guaco tea is typically taken orally. It can be consumed on its own or mixed with honey or other herbal teas for added flavor.

Side Effects: Guaco is generally considered safe for most people when used in moderate amounts. However, some individuals may experience allergic reactions or digestive upset. It may also interact with certain medications or have adverse effects in individuals with certain health conditions. It's important to use guaco under the guidance of a healthcare professional and to discontinue use if any adverse effects occur.

Bromide Plus Powder:

Definition: Bromide Plus Powder is a dietary supplement formulated to support thyroid health and promote overall well-being. It typically contains a blend of herbs and minerals that are believed to have beneficial effects on thyroid function.

Ingredients: Bromide Plus Powder often contains a combination of herbs such as bladderwrack, sea moss, and burdock root, along with minerals like iodine and potassium phosphate. These ingredients are thought to support thyroid function and maintain optimal iodine levels in the body.

How to Prepare: Bromide Plus Powder is usually mixed with water or juice to create a drinkable solution. It's important to follow the instructions on the product label for dosage and preparation.

Dosage: The dosage of Bromide Plus Powder can vary depending on the specific product and individual needs. It's crucial to consult with a healthcare professional or follow the recommended dosage on the product label to avoid potential side effects.

How to Use: Bromide Plus Powder is typically taken orally by mixing the recommended dosage with water or juice. It's important to shake or stir the mixture well before consuming it to ensure even distribution of the ingredients.

Side Effects: While Bromide Plus Powder is generally considered safe when used as directed, some individuals may experience side effects such as digestive discomfort or allergic reactions to certain ingredients. It's essential to consult with a healthcare provider before starting any new supplement regimen, especially if you have underlying health conditions or are taking medications.

Bugleweed:

Definition: Bugleweed, also known as Lycopusvirginicus, is a perennial herb native to North America and Europe. It has been used in traditional medicine to treat various conditions, including hyperthyroidism, anxiety, and insomnia.

Ingredients: Bugleweed contains several active compounds, including lithospermic acid, phenolic acids, and flavonoids. These compounds are believed to contribute to the herb's medicinal properties, particularly its ability to regulate thyroid function.

How to Prepare: Bugleweed is commonly consumed as a tea or tincture. To make tea, dried bugleweed leaves and flowers are steeped in hot water for several minutes before being strained and consumed. Tinctures are prepared by steeping the herb in alcohol or vinegar to extract its active compounds.

Dosage: The appropriate dosage of bugleweed can vary depending on factors such as age, health status, and the specific preparation being used. It's important to follow the recommended dosage on the product label or consult with a qualified herbalist or healthcare professional for personalized guidance.

How to Use: Bugleweed tea or tincture is typically taken orally. It can be consumed on its own or mixed with honey or other herbal teas for added flavor.

Side Effects: While bugleweed is generally considered safe for most people when used in moderation, excessive intake may cause digestive upset or allergic reactions in some individuals. Pregnant or breastfeeding women should avoid bugleweed due to its potential to stimulate uterine contractions. As with any herbal remedy, it's important to consult with a healthcare provider before using bugleweed, especially if you have underlying health conditions or are taking medications.

THE END